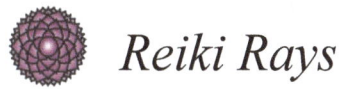

Reiki Rays

THE REIKI BOOKLET

Reiki Symbols, Hand Positions,
Archangels, and Chakras

Copyright

Reiki is not a replacement for medical assistance. Always seek professional medical support if you experience anything that requires it. Seek the services of a competent professional if expert assistance is required.

To fully understand and to be able to apply the techniques described in this book, the reader should already be introduced to the healing magic of Reiki.

Table of Contents

Reiki Symbols

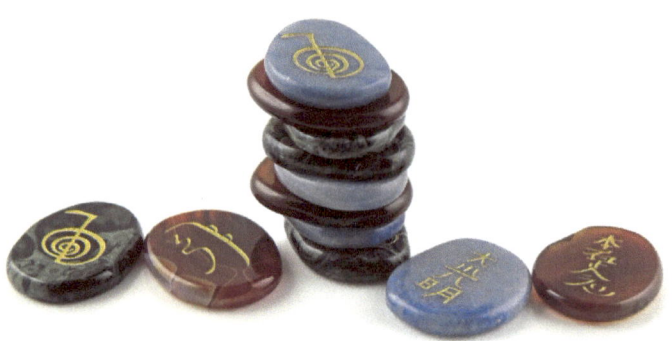

Drawing Reiki Symbols

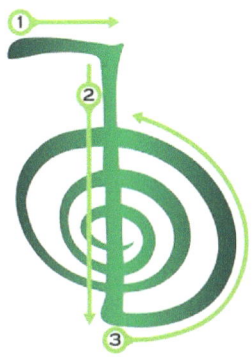

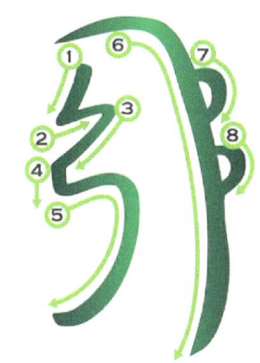

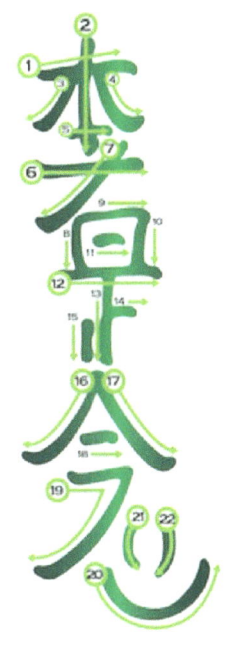

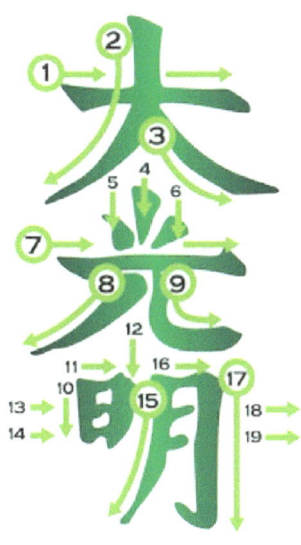

Cho Ku Rei - Power Symbol

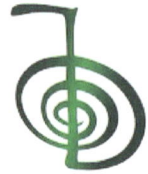

Meaning

"Placing all the powers of the universe here."

How to Use the Symbol

Used primarily to boost the Reiki power, to connect with Reiki energy at the start of a session, and to seal the energy at the end of a treatment.

Some practitioners use it on their own palms and chakras before treating others, to help clear the channels and empower their hands.

Using the power symbol over the client's Crown chakra helps create positive energy around them.

Example Uses

Empower other Reiki symbols
Helps in spot treatment
Clears negative energies
Provide protection

Makes meals healthier and more nutritious
Increase effectiveness and reduce side effects of medication
Improve relationships
Prevent misfortunes
Activate the law of attraction

Sei He Ki - Emotional / Mental Healing Symbol

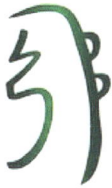

Meaning

"The earth and sky meet" or "God and Man become one."

How to Use the Symbol

Different practitioners use this symbol in different ways. As an example, the practitioner draws the Cho Ku Rei (the power symbol) to create a connection with the Reiki energy source. Sei He Ki is then drawn over the troubled area where the Reiki energies are required. The energies are sealed by drawing the power symbol again. This sustains the effect of Sei He Ki for a longer time.

Example Uses

Improve memory power
Get rid of bad habits
Improve relationships
Empowers your affirmations
Dissipates headaches

Helps to find lost objects
Teaches us about the synchronization or harmony of things in nature
Gain more positive outlook of life and stay happy

Hon Sha Ze Sho Nen - Distance Healing Symbol

Meaning

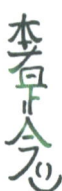

Having no present, past or future.

How to Use the Symbol

There are many ways to send Reiki. A lot of practitioners learn one technique, which they then tweak and personalize it to suite their style. The steps below describe one such technique:

1. Activate the power symbol.
2. Write the name of the recipient or the situation you are sending energy to on a piece of paper and hold the paper in between your hands.
3. Draw Hon Sha Ze Sho Nen in the air above the paper and repeat its name three times.
4. Repeat the name of the recipient or the situation. Draw the power symbol.
5. Allow Reiki to flow to the recipient for the greatest and highest good.
6. Finish the Reiki session by either clapping your hands or shaking them vigorously in order to cut the connection.

Example Uses

Allows sending and receiving positive energy just anywhere and everywhere quickly and easily

Perfect tool for people who find it uncomfortable to receive hands on Reiki treatment

Used regularly to help keep your mind, body and spirit in harmony

Healing the past

Sending positive energy to the future

Absentee healing

Dai Ko Myo - Master Symbol

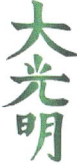

Meaning

"Great Enlightenment" or "Bright Shining Light."

How to Use the Symbol

The symbol can be activated in many ways, including but not limited to:

Drawing it on your palm center by visualizing it
Drawing the symbol with your finger
Drawing it with your Third Eye
Spelling the name of the symbol three times.

Example: First draw the Reiki symbol on your own palms or hands and then visualize or redraw the symbol on the Crown chakra and the palms or hands of the client and the area to be treated.

Example Uses

Open channels during Reiki attunement
Heals the chakras, the aura and any disease that initiates from our subconscious beliefs
Draw out negative energy from the body (physical, emotional, mental or spiritual) and then liberate it
Develop and strengthen personal growth, self-awareness, spiritual development and intuition
To charge or clear crystals
Helps improve immune function and increase energy flow through the body.

Hands Positions

Hand Positions for Self Treatment

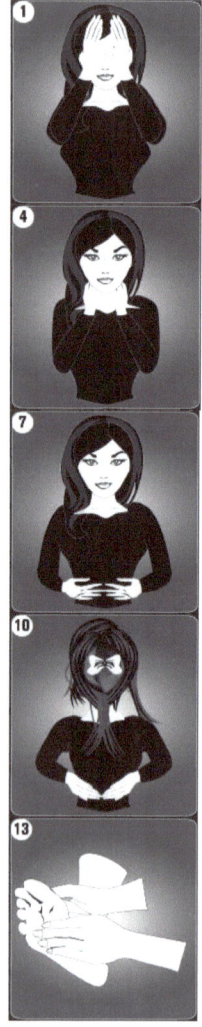
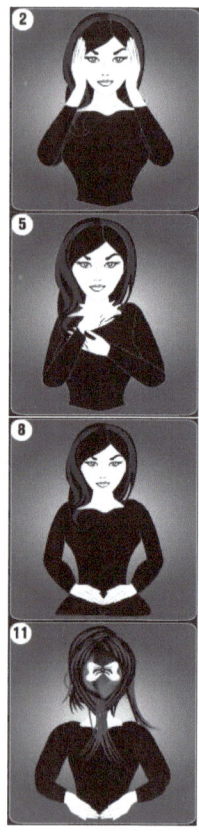
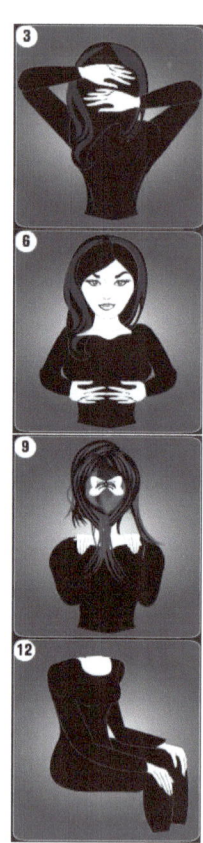

Reiki Hand Positions
for self-treatment
Reiki Rays © 2013
http://reikirays.com

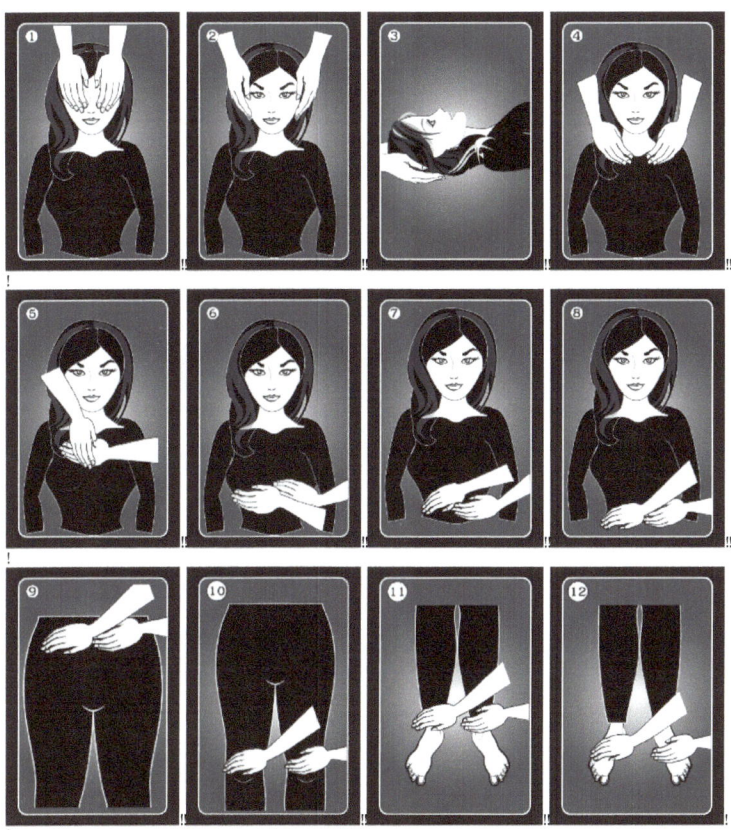

Reiki Hand Positions
for healing others
Reiki Rays © 2014
http://reikirays.com

Archangels

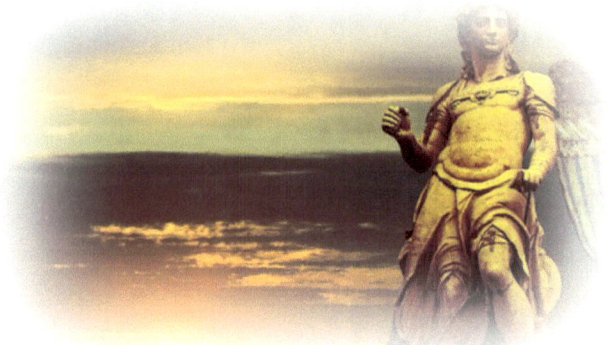

Archangel Michael - "Who is Like God"

In charge of Protection, Justice, Truth.

Color - Royal purple that's so bright, it looks like cobalt blue.

Call when in need

If you find yourself under psychic attack.

When your job is too demanding or impossible.

When you have deadlines to reach and people to handle.

Reiki Symbol

Dai Ko Myo - Master Symbol

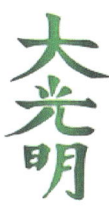

Archangel Gabriel - "Messenger of God"

In charge of Communication.

Color - White and purple light.

Call when in need

If your Third Eye is closed.

If you want a child she may help you conceive or bring news of conception.

Very helpful for women who have been abused.

To stay on life path and to know soul's plan.

Reiki Symbol

Cho Ku Rei - Power Symbol

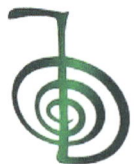

Archangel Raphael - "God heals"

In charge of Love, Miracles, Grace.

Color - Green light.

Call when in need

When you are traveling.

When you need to heal from physical, emotional and mental pain.
Heal wounds from past lives & childhood trauma.

Finding lost pets and even lost soul mates.
Can help in marriages.

Reiki Symbol

Sei He Ki – Emotional / Mental Healing Symbol

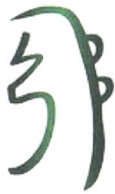

Archangel Uriel - "The Light of God"

In charge of Transformation, Transmutation.

Color - Golden light.

Call when in need

Heals all natural calamities.

Heals the Earth.

When you need to release the painful burdens and memories of the past.

Reiki Symbol

Hon Sha Ze Sho Nen – Distance Healing Symbol

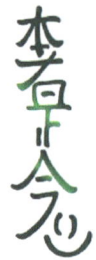

Chakras

● Crown Chakra
● Brow Chakra

● Throat Chakra

● Heart Chakra

● Solar Plexus Chakra

● Sacral Chakra
● Root Chakra

Crown Chakra

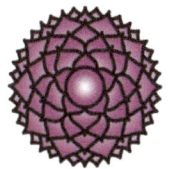

Color - Violet

Location - Top of the head

Associated Organs and Glands - Brain, nervous system, pituitary gland

Chakra Test

Balanced	Overactive	Underactive
Joy Connected to "the Source" while aware of one's individuality Wise Compassionate	Addicted to spirituality Craving attention Needing to be popular Over-erotic imagination	Misunderstood Can't have fun Unaware of or denying one's spiritual connection

Brow Chakra - Third Eye

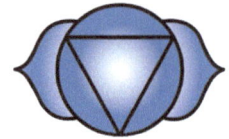

Color - Indigo

Location - Above the eyes, center of the forehead

Associated Organs and Glands - Pineal gland, eyes, nose, ears, skeletal system

Chakra Test

Balanced	Overactive	Underactive
Intuitive Charismatic Can meditate Knows one's purpose Seen as wise	Spaced out Lost Worrying Seen as living in a fantasy world	Can't see the bigger picture Can be easily influenced Confused about one's purpose Doubting oneself

Throat Chakra

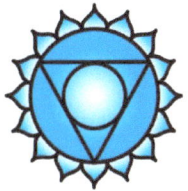

Color - Blue

Location - Base of the throat

Associated Organs and Glands - Thyroid gland, larynx, trachea, ears, nose, teeth, mouth, throat, carotid arteries

Chakra Test

Balanced	Overactive	Underactive
Can express self Speaks truth Creative	Speaking too much Boring others Seen as criticizing Stubborn	Can't express self Afraid to speak in public Cannot express the creative side Seen as timid Dependent

Heart Chakra

Color - Green

Location - Heart, center of the chest

Associated Organs and Glands - Circulatory system (including heart), respiratory system, arms, hands, shoulders, ribs, breasts, diaphragm, and thymus gland

Chakra Test

Balanced	Overactive	Underactive
Loved Loving Empathetic "Contagiously" good vibe	Entitlement Jealousy Blaming others Giving too much	Unloved Self pity Fear of rejection Neediness Clinginess Uncertainty

Solar Plexus Chakra

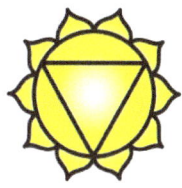

Color - Yellow

Location - Between the sternum and the navel

Associated Organs and Glands - Nervous system, stomach, gall bladder, large intestine, liver, and pancreas

Chakra Test

Balanced	Overactive	Underactive
Respect for self and others Confident Outgoing Problem solving Calm Integrity	Judgmental Stubborn Critical Bully	Low self esteem Apathetic Procrastinating "Taken advantage of" Not knowing what to do

Sacral Chakra

Color - Orange

Location - Lower abdomen, 1-2 inches below the navel

Associated Organs and Glands - Lymphatic and circulatory system, kidneys, adrenals, skin, female reproductive organs

Chakra Test

Balanced	Overactive	Underactive
Friendly Passionate Sexually fulfilled Good mood Playful Naturally flirty	Need power Manipulative Craving	Shy Guilty Afraid to interact Lost Overly concerned about what others think

Root Chakra

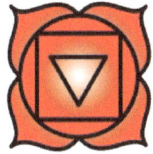

Color - Red

Location - Tailbone, base of the spine

Associated Organs and Glands - Spine, bladder, blood, kidneys, male reproductive organs, vagina, legs, feet

Chakra Test

Balanced	Overactive	Underactive
Grounded Centered Belonging in this world Trusting Independent Alive Poised	Bossy Domineering Big ego Greedy Violent Cunning	Unloved Sexually inadequate Frustrated Fearful Shy Unsure

Chakra Test

Symbol	Balanced	Overactive	Underactive
Crown Chakra	Joy Connected to "the Source" while aware of one's individuality Wise Compassionate	Addicted to spirituality Craving attention Needing to be popular Over-erotic imagination	Misunderstood Can't have fun Unaware of or denying one's spiritual connection
Brow Chakra (Third Eye)	Intuitive Charismatic Can meditate Knows one's purpose Seen as wise	Spaced out Lost Worrying Seen as living in a fantasy world	Can't see the bigger picture Can be easily influenced Confused about one's purpose Doubting oneself
Throat Chakra	Can express self Speaks truth Creative	Speaking too much Boring others Seen as criticizing Stubborn	Can't express self Afraid to speak in public Cannot express the creative side Seen as timid Dependent
Heart Chakra	Loved Loving Empathetic "Contagiously" good vibe	Entitlement Jealousy Blaming others Giving too much	Unloved Self pity Fear of rejection Neediness Clinginess Uncertainty
Solar Plexus Chakra	Respect for self and others Confident Outgoing Problem solving Calm Integrity	Judgmental Stubborn Critical Bully	Low self esteem Apathetic Procrastinating "Taken advantage of" Not knowing what to do
Sacral Chakra	Friendly Passionate Sexually fulfilled Good mood Playful Naturally flirty	Need power Manipulative Craving	Shy Guilty Afraid to interact Lost Overly concerned about what others think
Root Chakra	Grounded Belonging in this world Trusting Independent Alive Poised	Bossy Domineering Big ego Greedy Violent Cunning	Unloved Sexually inadequate Frustrated Fearful Shy Unsure

The Five Reiki Principles

Just for today…Do not anger

Just for today…Do not worry

Just for today…Be grateful for your many blessings

Just for today…Work honestly

Just for today…Be kind to all living things

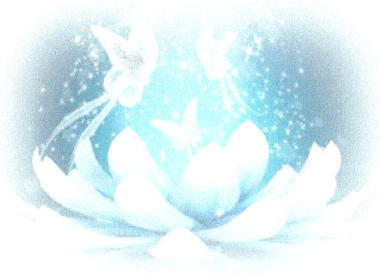

Love and Light!